APPLE CIDER
VINEGAR
SOLUTION

Discover the Many Miraculous Apple Cider
Vinegar Cures, Uses and Remedies You
Never Knew About

Sandi Lane

Limits of Liability, Disclaimer of Warranties & Terms of Use

This book is a general educational information product. As an express condition to reading this book, you understand and agree to following terms. The information and advice contained in this book are not intended as a substitute for consulting with a professional.

The publisher and author make no representations or warranties with respect to the accuracy or completeness of the contents of this work and specifically disclaim all warranties, including without limitation warranties of fitness for a particular purpose. No warranty may be created or extended by sales or promotional materials. The advice and strategies contained herein may not be suitable for every situation. This work is sold with the understanding that the publisher is not engaged in rendering legal, accounting, of the professional services. If professional assistance is required, the services of a competent professional person should be sought. Neither the publisher nor author shall be liable for damages arising therefrom.

ISBN-10: 1507553382
ISBN- 13: 978-1507553381

DEDICATION

This book is dedicated to those in search of the many uses and healing power of Apple Cider Vinegar.

CONTENTS

Introduction   i

1   What is Apple cider vinegar?   1

2   Benefits to Overall Health   5

3   ACV for Weight Loss   13

4   Skin Care, Hair Care and Oral Care   15

5   How Long Before you See Effects?   21

6   Other uses for Apple Cider Vinegar   25

INTRODUCTION

Have you ever wonder what miracle cures lie in your home for various illnesses? You may want to consider purchasing a bottle of apple cider vinegar the next time you're in the store. It may surprise you how versatile and beneficial this inexpensive vinegar is. Apple cider vinegar contains various vitamins and minerals, and has many health benefits.

This book contains proven steps and strategies on how to improve your overall health using Apple Cider Vinegar (ACV). It also has useful information on how to use ACV for your skin, hair, and oral care.

CHAPTER 1 – WHAT IS APPLE CIDER VINEGAR?

You must have heard about Apple cider vinegar (ACV) from friends, neighbors, people who have tried it and swear by its benefits. But, what is so special about it? After all, vinegar is vinegar right? So, before I start telling you about all the beneficial things that it can do for you; let's talk about what Apple cider vinegar is.

As the name implies, it comes from apples and, organic apples are the best to use when making Apple cider vinegar. If you're unsure (or really want organic stuff) you can make some at home. How? Well, you start with apples, cut into pieces and covered in water and left to ferment. The first result is what's called hard cider, and then you let it ferment again and then you get vinegar. Fermentation is the process used to turn other fruits and vegetables into vinegar. It is this process that allows the sugars in the apples to turn into alcohol.

There are many kinds of Apple cider vinegar that can be found in markets, but the best kind is the unpasteurized, unfiltered version—yes there are filtered and pasteurized kinds in the market and it is recommend looking for the one that has a murky consistency with sediments that settle in the bottom of the bottle. This is the best kind because you get loads more nutrients and enzymes from this kind.

Pasteurization is an old method used in preservation where the product is heated using very high heat and then cooled really quickly before storage. It allows liquid products like milk to remain fresh for longer periods of time.

Why is it not good for Apple cider vinegar? Heating removes many of its health benefits; for one thing, pasteurization will remove Mycoderma aceti, also known as Mother of vinegar. This is a substance that contains acetic acid; it is what turns the alcohol produced from the fermented apples into acetic acid. This is the healthiest part of ACV, and later on you will learn about the many things it can do for you.

Pasteurization will also remove its murky appearance. Sure, it looks good, but the reason you bought Apple cider vinegar (as opposed to buying regular vinegar) is because of its many health benefits it comes with, right? The murky, amber color and the sediments at the bottom are what you want from this product. You have to make sure that whenever you use this to shake it well so that the sediments that have settled at the bottom will mix with the whole solution again so you get all the goodness.

You would also want an organic Apple cider vinegar as opposed to a distilled one. Most of the time, organic ACV has been fermented using wood barrels that add additional benefits to the product as it helps in the natural fermentation process. Whereas distilled variants may not have the same benefits. Again, the appearance of the organic, non-distilled, unpasteurized Apple cider vinegar may not be pleasing to eyes, but believe me, it has all the good stuff.

Sandi Lane

CHAPTER 2 – BENEFITS TO OVERALL HEALTH

Apple cider vinegar is a healthy alternative as opposed to regular white vinegar. Here are more reasons why you should choose ACV instead:

Acetic acid is an organic compound that gives it that very distinct sour taste and really strong, pungent smell. It is also packed with anti-microbial properties that kill certain types of bacteria, including E.coli. It inhibits the formation of more bacteria, too.

Remember the sediments that settle at the bottom of the bottle (again, you only get this with unpasteurized, organic Apple cider vinegar), that is also known as the mother of vinegar and it comes packed with probiotics. What are probiotics? These are good bacteria that you have, naturally, in your digestive tract. These friendly bacteria help boost the immune system, and help with bowel movement. So, if you're constipated or have an irritable bowel movement, drinking Apple cider vinegar can alleviate some (if not all) of that discomfort. Regular intake of ACV will more or less regulate your bowel movement and help keep your digestive tract healthy.

Detoxification, Allergies and Heartburn

Another health benefit you get from Apple cider vinegar is detoxification. It not only removes toxins from your digestive tract, but it also detoxifies your liver. It also blocks some of the starch from your food, preventing it from raising the sugar level of your blood. If you eat starchy food, the excess starch that your body doesn't digest will then become food for the good bacteria in your body. It has an anti-glycemic effect that has been proven to be very beneficial especially to people suffering from diabetes.

It even improves insulin function; for example, while you eat foods high in carbohydrates, Apple cider vinegar improves insulin sensitivity allowing your body to process the sugars in the food before they settle into your bloodstream. While it does not claim to be a cure for diabetes, it is still a very helpful and healthy product diabetics can use to help them with the disease.

People who suffer from allergies will also benefit from Apple cider vinegar because it breaks out mucus in your body and it also cleans the lymph nodes and alleviate sinus congestion and, because it has anti-bacterial and anti-fungal properties, Apple cider vinegar can fend off infections and related symptoms that cause headaches or sore throat.

If you are suffering from acid-reflux or heartburn, you can also use Apple cider vinegar to alleviate this. I know it sounds weird—treating acid with acid—but what Apple cider vinegar does is it balances the low acids which causes heartburn. With a balanced out amount of low acids, you don't get acid-reflux. (This will not work if you have ulcers, though, so please do not use this to treat ulcers).

Heart and Cholesterol

Another health benefit that is important to mention, is how it helps the heart. Heart disease and stroke are the world's leading (if not one of the major) causes of death. A major cause of heart disease and even stroke would be having high cholesterol levels—LDL or Low-density lipoprotein, also known as the bad cholesterol, and is the kind that causes heart diseases.

It becomes even more dangerous when it comes into contact with free-radicals because this causes the LDL cholesterol to get oxidized. Oxidized LDL cholesterol can cause tissue damage, and they accumulate in the arteries that supply blood to your extremities and heart. Once there, they will promote inflammatory cells that will accumulate along with platelets and other lipids. This, in turn, becomes plaque and piles up causing blockage in the arteries.

Apple cider vinegar contains an antioxidant called chlorogenic acid that is known to shield LDL (Low-density lipoprotein) cholesterol from being oxidized. The process of oxidation of LDL cholesterol has been alluded as the first step to heart disease. So, preventing this from happening will lower down the risk. There's also proof that Apple cider vinegar lowers blood pressure.

Sooth Pain and Boost Energy

ACV can also be used to soothe aches and pains. You can use it like a balm or massage lotion. The acetic acid gives a warm feeling that is good when used topically for soothing aching muscles and joints.

Lastly, Apple cider vinegar also has potassium and enzymes that can boost your energy levels. If you need a pick-me-upper, skip the energy drinks and instead mix up a glass of Apple cider vinegar and water (you can even add honey to make it taste better) and, voila. You have an instant energy-boosting drink that is all natural. It also has amino acids that help fight off fatigue, so if you're feeling tired, or really bummed out, and you need your energy level to go up, mix up some of this concoction and see yourself come back to life.

Increasing the potassium level in your body not only helps with the energy boost, but also with leg cramps. If you also suffer from nighttime restless leg syndrome, Apple cider vinegar can help you with that, too.

It has also been discovered that you can use Apple cider vinegar to treat kidney stones. Apart from helping you cope with the pain that comes with having kidney stones, Apple cider vinegar can also break up the kidney stones because of the citric acid in it. This citric acid will soften the stones and make it easier for the body to flush it out. And, because it is acidic, it can help dissolve crystals that form into stones in your body (so you prevent the stones from ever becoming a problem with constant ingestion of Apple cider vinegar). Apple cider vinegar also has phosphoric acid that reduces the size of kidney stones (and in some cases, dissolve them completely) so you can pass them freely through the urethra.

Women's Health

For women, Apple cider vinegar can also be used to alleviate vaginal irritation. This is a problem not only because it is very uncomfortable, but it is also very embarrassing. While vaginal irritation can be cause by many factors like yeast infection, chemical irritation from vaginal washes or menstrual pads or panty liners, tight clothing, lack of personal hygiene, or other reasons, one thing is certain—when it persists, it can become really painful. A severe infection in your genital area can lead to other more serious problems, so before it does, we highly recommend to see a doctor of course to address this. In the meantime, you can use Apple cider vinegar to help you cope with the itch. You see, Apple cider vinegar has anti-bacterial and anti-fungal properties.

Most vaginal irritations are caused by bacteria or fungi, so washing your vaginal area with Apple cider vinegar water solution will dramatically help in completely removing the itchiness and lower down the inflammation of the skin. You can even make Apple cider vinegar ice cubes and use it to soothe the itchy skin. The cold sensation will definitely have an immediate soothing effect on the irritated skin as the Apple cider vinegar works its way, killing the bacteria and fungus.

Now, if you are a woman going through menopause or have gone through it, you are familiar with all its symptoms. They can range from the uncomfortable to the downright maddening. You can use Apple cider vinegar to relieve per-menopausal and menopausal symptoms like night sweats and hot flashes.

Apple cider vinegar helps keep your bones healthy because it has calcium. It also decreases the progression of osteoporosis because it has magnesium and manganese. Apple cider vinegar also helps your body absorb minerals and nutrients easier and faster from the food you eat because again, it helps digestion.

Gout and Arthritis

Speaking of bones, another problem that can be eased by drinking Apple cider vinegar is gout and arthritis. The cause of these debilitated healthy issues is an imbalance in your body's acid level—which leads to acidosis, and this is the root of many diseases. When your body's pH level goes haywire, your body will try to fix itself will result in high uric acid levels that cause muscle spasms. So, normalizing the pH level of your body is important.

Apple cider vinegar helps your body by stimulating important digestive juices, like bicarbonate (which is an alkaline release by the pancreas). This alkaline neutralizes the acids in your stomach and, thus, brings your body's pH level back to its normal state. With your body in balance, it won't try to balance out itself and produce uric acid that results in rheumatic gout.

Apple cider vinegar also helps you cope with the pain caused by gout and arthritis.

Another thing that Apple cider vinegar can help you with is for curing toenail fungus. You get toenail fungus if you have a weak immune system and your feet is always in sweaty shoes (that are probably full of bacteria), or simply lack of personal hygiene. Because of its anti-bacterial and anti-fungal properties, it is the best natural remedy for toenail infections due to fungus.

So, when you start seeing yellow toenails, or discoloration, swelling and cracking—you should start your Apple cider vinegar solution routine. Mix equal parts of Apple cider vinegar and water and soak your infected toenail for at least half an hour. Then, use Apple cider vinegar to clean and disinfect your shoes so that any bacteria in it will die and not get your other toenails infected.

Sandi Lane

CHAPTER 3 – ACV FOR WEIGHT LOSS

Here's a fact: toxins make you fat and keep you fat. So, anything that will help detoxify your body will definitely help you lose weight. As we have discussed in an earlier chapter, Apple cider vinegar helps keep your digestive system healthy with the probiotics—or good bacteria—and it also helps keep your liver healthy.

The liver's main function is to filter the blood and liquids you put into your body. A healthy liver means good detoxification of harmful waste products that not only inhibit weight loss, but promote diseases. So, in that aspect alone, Apple cider vinegar is already a great agent in inducing weight-loss.

Another thing it does is it lowers your craving for sugary foods. If you like eating sweets, or carbohydrate-filled foods, you know that most of it doesn't get processed and end up as stored fat in your body. Apple cider vinegar helps flush out carbohydrates like it does fiber. It just goes through you system without being stored as fat, and it also trims down water retention.

We also said that Apple cider vinegar gives you energy,

especially if you drink it first thing in the morning, it will perk you up and give you that much needed boost to do more exercise. We all know that weight loss is difficult if you're only cutting down on food intake. You need to move. You need to do exercise to really burn stored fat, and having lots of energy will help you do just that.

It also helps alkalize the body. What does that do? Our bodies produce acid and anything that produces acid or is in an acidic state harbors disease-causing bacteria to form. Alkalizing the body will neutralize that.

It also helps boost your immune system so you stay on top of your game all the time. When you get sick, it takes a while for the body to get back to its fighting form, and, normally we sleep more and eat more when we are sick to compensate for the body's weak state.

Though it's true that some people lose weight when they get sick, it is also true that there are those who gain weight while they are sick and soon after. They believe that since you just got better you should take it easy. Unfortunately, this kind of attitude can extend sometimes, and you forget the whole reason why you're exercising. So, a good immune system will get rid of all that. You stay healthy enough to stick to your regimen and, in no time, you will get that killer body you've always dreamed of.

If you ever have that bloated feeling—just drink a glass of water with two tablespoons of Apple cider vinegar and it will be relieved.

CHAPTER 4- SKIN CARE, HAIR CARE AND ORAL CARE

This may come as a surprise because of course it's vinegar. You probably have doubts and inhibitions about using vinegar on your skin. For one thing, the smell—it is definitely not the usual facial product smell. However, it has been tested and proven effective. Here are a few of the remedies it does for your skin.

Apple cider vinegar can clear acne—yes, you read it right, it clears acne. Of course, it is not recommended that you use Apple cider vinegar directly onto your face. It is still vinegar and can therefore burn your skin. However, because of its acetic acid content, and anti-bacterial and anti-inflammatory agents, it is perfect to use when mixed with other organic skin care products for your face.

For example, you can dilute two tablespoons of Apple cider vinegar in rosewater (or rosewater glycerin) and make yourself a homemade organic toner. This gets rid of all the impurities in your skin and kills bacteria at the same time.

Also, if you have breakouts, the anti-inflammatory agent will lower down inflammation in the skin and in no time at all, the acne would dry up and be cured.

With its lactic and malic acid content, it is perfect for sloughing off dead skin. We all know that dead skin cells are the favorite food of bacteria which, causes acne. So, by removing the smorgasbord from your face, you are technically starving the bacteria, and then in comes the anti-bacterial agents again to kill them off completely. It also helps to balance out the pH level of your skin to give you that vibrant, healthy glow. Apple cider vinegar can even be used as an organic after-shave.

You can also use Apple cider vinegar for your bruises. The anti-inflammatory properties of Apple cider vinegar will lower down the swelling, and help the discoloration to go away.

Apple cider vinegar can soothe the itchiness caused by jellyfish stings, poison ivy, and insect bites. Another thing Apple cider vinegar can do is to help remove body odor. Yes, you can use Apple cider vinegar because it also has anti-fungal properties. You can use it to deodorize your feet and other smelly body parts. Since it balances pH levels in your skin, it works against bacteria that cause body odor. Again, you don't have to apply Apple cider vinegar directly onto skin, you can dilute it in water and use a spray bottle or use a moist towel or a baby wipe.

You can also use Apple cider vinegar to treat sunburns. Add some Apple cider vinegar to your bath water and turn it into a soothing spa for your sun-burnt skin.

Now, for pesky warts, you can use Apple cider vinegar as treatment. Dip a cotton swab in Apple cider vinegar and dab directly onto the wart. Leave it overnight. This will have a stinging sensation, but that's okay, that's how you know it's working.

You can also use Apple cider vinegar to get rid of raised moles. Of course, make sure first that the said mole is benign and not malignant before you do anything to it. So, consult a doctor and find out if that mole is safe to remove.

If it is, then you can abrade it sufficiently so that it allows the Apple cider vinegar to penetrate the mole and kill it. Soak the mole overnight with Apple cider vinegar and the next day, wash up and you will see that the mole will start to look like a scab. What it did is it burned your mole and now it is dead and ready to be sloughed off.

Hair Care

Anything that is good for skin should be good for your scalp too. Now, a major problem for a lot people is dealing with dandruff. There are many products in the market for dandruff control or cure. Apple cider vinegar is one of them. Since it balances the pH levels of your skin, you can also use it to do the same thing for your scalp.

A balanced pH level in your scalp will prevent the growth of yeast, which is the cause of dandruff. It also helps alleviate some of the things that come with dandruff like itchiness and irritation. It also helps remove the greasiness of your scalp. And so, adding Apple cider vinegar to your rinsing water will help clear your head of those pesky flakes.

Another thing it does for your hair is promoting healthy hair growth. Now, this, a lot of people may not believe, but, yes, you can use Apple cider vinegar to treat the problem of hair loss There are many solutions advertised to help promote hair growth and , but most are chemically induced and are quite expensive. Apple cider vinegar presents a healthy, organic way of keeping your hair growing and preventing you from losing too much.

Our hair needs nutrients to stay healthy, especially potassium, which is important for healthy hair growth. Now, as we have mentioned in previous chapters, Apple cider vinegar is rich in potassium that is good for boosting your energy levels, but it has also been proven to help boost your hair's health. It also has a lot of healthy enzymes and nutrients that keep your hair healthy. So, if you have healthy hair and a healthy scalp, hair loss will become a thing of the past.

Now, if your hair has been damaged by hair products like shampoos or treatments like perming or straightening, or just through overexposure to the sun, normally you will need different products to fix the damage in your hair, or you can use Apple cider vinegar to repair it. Yes, Apple cider vinegar also repairs damaged hair.

What it does is it restores that protective layer in your hair that you normally lose when you abuse your hair. This layer gets depleted whenever you get treatments that use harsh chemicals. You can even remove it by just by over shampooing your hair or using heat styling too often. People who love going to the beach can tell you that their hair has been severely damaged and this was because of so much exposure to the sun. Your hair should not be exposed to too much sunlight because the UV rays of the sun are really harmful to the hair strands. The sun will burn away that protective layer your hair badly needs to stay healthy.

Apple cider vinegar will help bring that layer back, and since it also cleans your scalp of all the gunk in it, it allows your hair to breathe freely, naturally.

So, using Apple cider vinegar to care for your hair is highly recommended. Apple cider vinegar will not only rejuvenate dry, damaged hair, prevent hair loss, and dandruff, but it also improves the quality of your hair.

Oral Care

We mentioned that Apple cider vinegar can soothe sore throat and that is because of its anti-bacterial properties that kill the germs that cause sore-throat. The same anti-bacterial properties will work well for other parts of your mouth. For instance, you can use Apple cider vinegar water as a gargle. Since it kills bacteria, it is a great product to use to get rid of bad breath. Make sure to dilute it in water before using it as a mouthwash as it can also be harsh on the gums.

Now, if you are also a person that suffers from yellow teeth, you can use Apple cider vinegar as a natural whitening agent. It will remove stubborn, hard-to-remove stains in your teeth that could have been caused by coffee or smoking.

To use Apple cider vinegar to whiten your teeth, use a cotton swab. Dip it in the Apple cider vinegar and rub the swab on your teeth then rinse with water. A note of caution though: do not do this on a daily basis since the acid in the Apple cider vinegar can break the enamel in your teeth. Maybe use this once or twice a month.

Sandi Lane

CHAPTER 5 – HOW LONG BEFORE YOU SEE EFFECTS?

Now that you know what Apple cider vinegar can do for you, I bet you're thinking about this next question: how soon before I begin to see any results? Especially if you're planning to use Apple cider vinegar for weight-loss, you may be anxious to see the effects as soon as possible. Who wouldn't?

I mean, anyone trying this out to get into that sexy physique as soon as possible, will be thinking "when is this going to happen?" and probably stop after a while if they don't see immediate results. Or if you're using this to cure your acne and get that beautiful, radiant skin that it's supposed to give, when's that happening? So, yes, people will be looking for immediate results and it's understandable because we all want something to work.

This is probably the reason why there are so many myths and urban legends about Apple cider vinegar going around. Well, some of those have been proven to be true, but, while all of us want a quick solution to our health problems, unfortunately, there isn't one, not even Apple cider vinegar can do such miracles. It does work, there are people who have tested it and it worked for them, so there's no reason why it won't work for you, but it will take time. You have to be patient as well as diligent with your regimen to make sure that you achieve your goal. Keep up with the program, as they say, and you will see results.

This goes the same for all the other health benefits that it promises, whether by drinking Apple cider vinegar or by applying it externally—all of this will require the aid of time and perseverance on your part.

For example, if you want to use Apple cider vinegar for you digestive tract, your liver, your skin, hair, and for oral care, just continue using it and all of those problems will be addressed in time. However, what you need to consider is the continuity of your routine—as long as you are able to continue adding some Apple cider vinegar to your daily routine, you will see results and these are good, lasting results.

There was even an experience where an overweight person tried to use Apple cider vinegar for weight-loss and, after four months, only lost two pounds. This is not a significant amount of weight-loss and to anyone who has been trying for a long time; this may come as a disappointment.

However, part of losing weight is not only what you put in your body, but how much of it you burn. So, don't put the weight of all your efforts on Apple cider vinegar. You have to use this in combination with other things like exercise and eating proper, healthy foods, too.

What we are trying to say is that there are no shortcuts

to this, but continuously using Apple cider vinegar will get you the results you want and expect.

Sandi Lane

CHAPTER 6 – OTHER USES FOR APPLE CIDER VINEGAR

So, what else is Apple cider vinegar good for? Well, it is perfect for making salad dressings for that oh so healthy veggie salad. Or you can use Apple cider vinegar just to add a good zing to your soups and strews. You can even use this to jazz up some of your baked goodies.

You can also use this to care for your pets. Everyone knows that the biggest problem with pets is fleas. Apple cider vinegar can be used as a bathing solution to help keep fleas away from our furry family members. What you can do is mix a little Apple cider vinegar with water and, the first method of usage for this is to use it as a kind of rub for the severely infected areas of their fur. Massage it into the fur until you work your way into their skin. This solution should be equal parts of water to Apple cider vinegar. After that, you can either leave the rub in their fur for a few minutes to allow the solution to work its magic, or you can rinse your pet's fur also using water with a little Apple cider vinegar. In this solution, make sure there's more water than Apple cider vinegar. (Of course, we would still suggest that you consult your vet to find out if Apple cider vinegar is harmful to your pet or not).

Apple cider vinegar is also good as an all-purpose cleaner. It is a tried and tested mildew and mold killer for your shower curtains, but it can also be used as a disinfectant spray. Mix Apple cider vinegar with water (make this equal parts as well), and use a spray bottle to turn this into your own handy, homemade, organic, and really safe disinfectant spray. What it does is it helps clean surfaces and kills the bacteria in them, leaving them not just clean, but bacteria-free.

Apple cider vinegar also absorbs odor—yes, it has its own pungent smell, but that doesn't last long. In fact, after a while, it dissipates to nothing, which means, you can use your Apple cider vinegar also as an air freshener. So, it is a healthy, organic alternative to supermarket products that are made up of toxic chemicals.

So, use it to remove all the stinky smell in any room. Be it smoky smell from cooking fish or other smelly foods, to that weird smell in the bathroom, to that foot-smell in your bedroom. It does help get rid of body odor, which include foot-odor, too, so, you're not only getting rid of the source of that foot-smell (that really nasty, corn-chip smell), but you will also be able to get rid of whatever is left behind, if you know what I mean. So, goodbye smelly room, and say hello to fresh, clean, bacteria-free air.

Now, if there is a funky smell in a room that you just can't distinguish or remove topically (because maybe you can't find the source), don't worry. Just leave some Apple cider vinegar in a bowl and place it where the smell is the strongest and soon, that funky scent will disappear.

For those of you who are into gardening, listen up. You can also use Apple cider vinegar for your plants. As you grow your garden you can get rid of weeds

Please Leave a Review

Finally, if you enjoyed this book, please take the time to share your thoughts and post a review on Amazon. It would be greatly appreciated.

That review and feedback will help me improve the content in my books – and make each and every one more relevant and helpful to you.

Thank you again and good luck.

Sandi Lane

Made in United States
North Haven, CT
29 May 2022

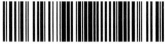

19645110R00022